WHAT WOULD FLO DO?

A REAL-WORLD GUIDE TO SURVIVING NURSING ORIENTATION

Rachel Edmondson, BHA, BSN, RN-BC

Cover created by Katie Swaim Design

Ordering Information
Quantity sales: Special discounts are available on quantity purchases by corporations, associations, and others. For details, contact the publisher at the above email address.

Printed in the United States of America.
ISBN 13: 978-0-9981114-2-1
ISBN 10: 0-9981114-2-2

Disclaimer
The information provided herein is stated to be truthful and consistent, in that any liability, in terms of inattention or otherwise, by any usage or abuse of any policies, processes, or directions contained within is the solitary and utter responsibility of the recipient reader. Under no circumstances will any legal responsibility or blame be held against the publisher for any reparation, damages, or monetary loss due to the information herein, either directly or indirectly.

The information herein is offered for informational purposes solely, and is universal as so. The presentation of the information is without contract or any type of guarantee assurance.

The trademarks that are used are without any consent, and the publication of the trademark is without permission or backing by the trademark owner. All trademarks and brands within this book are for clarifying purposes only and are owned by the owners themselves, not affiliated with this document.

CONTENTS

Hello Nurse Residents,

As the nurse managers of the residency program, we would like to formally welcome you to the Novant Health nursing team! Nursing leaders and team members have been looking forward to your arrival.

One of the main objectives of the nurse residency program is to help ease the transition into professional practice. This book is one resource that will provide insight as you begin this busy and exciting time. Every nurse can attest that one of the biggest milestones in your nursing journey is the successful completion of your orientation. Knowing what to expect will help you feel more confident as you enter into your orientation phase. By applying tips outlined in this book your residency journey will be off to a great start.

We are excited for you as you begin your nursing career. All of us at Novant Health look forward to supporting you every step of the way.

Traveling the residency road,

Lindsey Horne and Tracey Whitley

Managers of Nurse Residencies

INTRODUCTION

Everyone needs a tribe, an instinctual community, and a family with like purpose, bound together by common dialect, intention, and social likeness. We are Nurse Tribe. Our dialect is human touch and the power of medicine. Our purpose is the protection and healing of humankind. Our likeness, compassion, grace, and servitude.

Carefully curated to educate and inspire, Nurse Tribe offers a place of solitude, of connectedness, of raw, unfiltered (sometimes grammatically incorrect) candidness about navigating a world that misunderstands the magic of what we do. As an affiliate of Nurseology, an Austin-based company that sells products for nurses, Nurse Tribe seeks to connect and empower nurses through social media, e-publications, and online material.

> **Our Mission**
> Provide resources that draw on experience to further strengthen our tribe's fabric, to tighten our bond, and to bring to light
> the power of nursing.

1
OH, HEY THERE, SUNSHINE!

Look at you, stud. You've landed your first nursing job! The amount of blood, sweat, tears, laughter, joy, and heart palpitations that you endured to get where you are was no easy feat, but you did it. This leads me to believe you already have what it takes to not only survive your first baby nursing gig but to dominate it Bey' style. That's right, run the world.

So, here we are. You've already scoured the internet, downloaded the apps, and poured through Pinterest to find tips and tricks to surviving as a new grad nurse. You've read (and probably written down in your new planner) to drink lots of water and get 8 hours of sleep at night. Oh, don't forget to develop a mindful meditation practice, not take your code blue home with you, and decompress after you get off from work.

I know what you have found online and purchased because I was in your shoes several years ago. In fact, when I was writing this book, I searched the internet trying to see if the information out there had gotten even the slightest bit more helpful and real over the years. Sadly, the answer is no—even though the nursing world is constantly evolving.

Yes, friend, it is very important to stay hydrated and find time for yourself. One cannot negate these proven facts. Florence Nightingale has been dishing out this advice since 1854, but who is talking about how to give a quick, foolproof bedside shift report or unfreeze yourself during a code? Who is talking about how to sound like *you've-done-this-a-million-times-even-though-it's-your-first-time-SBAR* when you're STAT paging a doctor?

That would be me. Insert my name here: <u>Rachel</u>.

I have worked as a bedside nurse and precepted gaggles of baby nurses. I have played charge nurse, mediator, nurse's aid, lifesaver, hand-holder, bully-fighter, and nurse manager of a critical care unit. I ain't no Florence (lovingly referred to as "Flo" throughout this book), but I've earned some street cred in my few years of nursing. Regardless, I still make mistakes, get knocked down, and proudly admit I have more to learn.

Let me tell you what this book is *not*. This book is *not* perfect. It is *not* in strict APA format. You will find that some words, sentences, and punctuation are grammatically incorrect on purpose. I know my nursing professors are falling out of their chairs right now, buttttt I want you to imagine me talking to you in person, face to face, like the real person that I am. This is not a long manuscript that has all the answers to guarantee your nursing success, only you can do *that*.

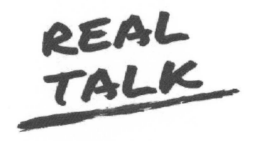

This book is candid and based on my real-life experiences, mistakes, and *wish-I-would-have-known-that* situations that have helped shape my nursing practice. It was written in an attempt to help you navigate the messy real world of nursing that is often sheepishly brushed over with the "drink lots of water" jargon. It is bulleted, starred, short, sweet, and to the point with a down-and-dirty perspective. My only hope is that it adequately prepares you for the rollercoaster that lies ahead and helps you reach Bey' status in a hurry.

2
THE BLIND DATE

Chances are that your organization will pair you with a preceptor whose schedule you will follow throughout your orientation. In some cases, if you are lucky, you will meet your preceptor before your first shift. However, most of you will meet your preceptor on your very first shift at a crazy weird hour.

Let's be clear: You. Will. Feel. Awkward. There is no doubt about it.

Frankly, you are a total stranger on your first blind date. It is early. Likely, no one has had their cup-o'-joe and your preceptor could resemble the grumpy cat meme more so than a human. Welcome to your first blind nursing date.

How to Deal
- Come to work about 30 minutes early. If you are told shift change starts at 0645, be on the unit between 0615 and 0630. You do not have to continue doing this, but being early on the first day is important.
- Find someone who looks like they own the place. You will likely pinpoint the charge nurse. Tell him it's your first day and ask him what to do next.
- Introduce yourself to your preceptor and begin to take note of what she is doing. How are the nurses determining who their patients are for the shift? What does the assignment sheet look like? What are they writing down?

Your preceptor will not bite, but do not bombard him with questions within the first 30 minutes of meeting him. Be present. Listen. Ask appropriate, simple questions.

3
YOUR FIRST SHIFT

So, you've gotten to work early and awkwardly have met your blind date for the next several months. Phew. That's over.

Every new nurse's first shift varies. Your organization may have you "shadow" your preceptor on the first day; others make you jump right in and take a full patient load. It all depends on where you work and how your orientation is facilitated by your clinical educator and preceptor.

Here's a simplified list of first shift dos and don'ts that apply regardless of where you work or what department you are in.

Do

- Find out how and where you will get your assignment each day.
- Find the break room and the staff bathrooms on the unit.
- Find the cafeteria and learn its business hours (very important).
- Make sure you have or find out how to get access to
  - Pyxis or ADC
  - Computer system
  - Electronic Medical Record
- Find your nutrition room and supply room and do a walk-through of each.
- Write down important numbers, and learn how to get hold of the charge nurse and unit secretary.

- Observe your preceptor's "flow" to get an idea of the routine on the floor. Take note of the following:
  - Approximately when your preceptor passes meds.
  - What seems to be the busiest hour.
  - When your preceptor charts.
  - If they pass meds then assess or vice versa.
  - When the docs do rounds.
- Learn the process should you have to call in sick. You are not invincible, and life does happen whether we want it to or not. It will be OK. I promise!
- Tell your preceptor how you learn (ya'll, this can save you a lot of heartache later). How do you learn best? You know this. Are you visual? Hands-on? Be professional and upfront about how you will be most successful. This will help guide your preceptor on how to tailor your orientation.
- Exchange numbers with your preceptor at the end of the shift. I promise this will come in handy.

Don't
- Expect anyone to know it's your first day. Go ahead and plan on introducing yourself to anyone and everyone while they stare at you blankly.
- Expect your preceptor to trust you with patients at first. You may have given insulin 100 times in nursing school, but, by golly, your preceptor did not know you nor did she work with you while you were in school! Out of safety for your patients, she will need to watch you and verify that you know how to do nursing tasks and med passes before letting you fly solo. Get over it.
- Be afraid to ask questions even if you think they are silly! You may not have had to hang an IV piggyback in nursing school, so ask your preceptor to show you how

to do it. The nurses that do not ask questions are the nurses who kill patients.

- Expect to leave work right at the end of your shift. There is no official clock-out time. You must safely pass off care to the oncoming nurse and ensure your patients' needs are met before leaving. *You are an RN managing human lives; this is not a movie theatre.*
- Not eat lunch. Period.
- Think you are above or better than the nursing assistants or techs. It is everyone's responsibility to ensure that every patient is fed, bathed, turned, cleaned, comfortable.

> **WWFD?**
> **(What Would Flo Do)?**
> She would probably tell you that the above are the fundamentals of nursing care. In fact, I am pretty sure at one point she straight up said that we are not above the work of an aid. It takes a village to keep our patients alive and well. Be a leader.

You got this. First day jitters will be over soon.

4
THE WEANING PROCESS

Your orientation will most likely take place over 2 to 3 months. Each organization, unit, and specialty has different nurse/patient ratios, which, in turn, creates different outlines for the orientation process.

Typically, your unit will pair you with a preceptor whose schedule you will follow during orientation. The goal is to increase your patient load over the orientation period until you are independent. This should happen organically toward the end of your orientation. We are tryin' to take you from Simba to the Lion King in less than 10 to 12 weeks, give or take a few.

Regardless of the unit that you start on, your preceptor should aim to wean you from her iron-tight grip as part of your growing process.

Here, we'll look at how the weaning process generally looks, assuming you have a 10-week orientation. Expect your preceptor to do the following.

Week 1: Verify everything, including your basic skills, do almost all menial tasks, catch you up when you are behind, take report, give report, call physicians, talk the most in patient rooms, prioritize for you, give you feedback.

Weeks 2 and 3: Assist you with things you have never done before, remind you of pending action items, let you take the reins in your patient rooms, let you pass

15

medications on your own (but may quiz you first), listen to you give and take report, guide you on how to pick up your pace, insist you page physicians (but will be right by when you are talking), help you plan out your phone call before you page, jump in when you are in over your head, give you feedback.

Weeks 4, 5, and 6: Assist you with things you have never done before, wait slightly longer to remind you of pending action items (testing your knowledge), allow you to fly *almost* solo in your patient rooms, expect you to page physicians without the preceptor being present, still discuss why you are paging physicians, help you navigate challenging situations, give you feedback.

Weeks 6, 7, and 8: Assist you with things you have never done before, let some of your pending noncritical to-dos be late so that you understand the cascade, expect you to fly solo in your patient rooms, expect you to page physicians without prompting, help you critically think through questions by not giving you the answers, give you feedback.

Weeks 8, 9, and 10: Assist you with things you have never done before, remind you of your priorities, expect you to take a full patient load and be the boss of patient care, give you feedback.

Your preceptors are not performing a disappearing act on you, nor are they being mean to you. They are strategically preparing you for the day when you get off orientation and they are no longer present to remind you that routine labs are collected at 0400. They should always jump in during emergencies, but you need to sink a little before you swim so you can learn.

5
REALITY SHOCK

During nursing school, the burden of patient advocacy, protection, and safety lies solely on the primary RN's license and secondarily on your clinical instructor's license. That's not to say you are permitted to practice carelessly, but it *does* take the *gravity* of responsibility away from the student nurse.

Practicing under your own license now requires you to manage the entire patient experience. Patients' lives and your license depend on it. In nursing school, you learned how to complete a 30-minute head-to-toe assessment on a patient. You now need to condense that to a 5-to-6 minute accurate patient assessment, pass medications, locate an IV pump, draw labs, chart, handle a crumping patient, and find a red Popsicle when only green are available for your patient. Yes, you read that correctly.

Now, multiply all that craziness by 2, 3, 4, 5, or even 6 patients. It ain't easy, friend.

Begin to shift your thinking toward efficiency. You are no longer operating in a perfect world with endless time and no responsibility. You now have precious little time and all the responsibility. Reality is a hard pill to swallow the first couple of months. If you learn to embrace the chaos and become an excellent strategist, you will be successful over time. Don't worry—there is a whole chapter on this later.

WWFD?

Flo would tell you not to forget what you learned in nursing school, and I second that. Hear! Hear! Patient safety, the 5 rights of medication administration, compassionate care, therapeutic communication, and pathophysiology are the fundamentals of nursing that Flo has been preaching all of these years.

6
HAVE-TO-KNOWS

Over the next few months, your brain will be in overdrive. There is no doubt about this. You will learn things and forget things. You will be reminded of things and coached on things. You will make mistakes and not know the answers to many questions you are asked. All of these things are OK and part of the growing process.

Right out of the gate, friend, you must always know 2 things about your patients regardless of where you work. Write them down so that should an emergency arise, you always have this information handy.

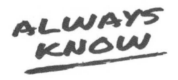

1. Your patients' code status. Always. Always. Always. If they are DNR or AND with interventions, you need to know what those interventions are. Intubation? Chest compressions? Antiarrhythmics? BIPAP? Temporary pacer?

2. Your patients' vital signs. Always. Always. Always. Vital signs can tell you so much about your patient. They are vital to your patient assessment, hence the term *vital signs*. Blood glucose is the 6th vital sign. The end. Neuro change? Diaphoresis? Altered Mental Status? Check their blood glucose.

19

7
PATIENT ASSESSMENT

I have said this before, and I will say it again before this book is over: *Your patient assessment is the single most important thing you will do all shift.* It should be concise and focused—it could save your patient's life.

If you work in a unit with telemetry monitoring capabilities, listen to me very carefully: Technology. Fails. All. The. Time.

I do not care if a patient's monitor says he is in sinus rhythm. Have you laid your hands on your patient and felt for a pulse? When you touch your patient and feel a pulse, you can feel if it's weak, thready, irregular, or normal. What if you can't feel a pulse, but the monitor shows a rhythm? It's called PEA arrest, nurse friend.

Always touch your patients. I learned this the hard way.

I know you are new, and feel like you don't know anything. That is 100% normal, but it is simply not true. Your nursing "gut" will tell you wonders. Even if you cannot put your finger on it, and the patient "just doesn't look right," go tell someone. If you follow your gut and use your senses, you will never fail.

> **WWFD?**
> Look. Touch. Feel. Smell. Listen.
> Do. Not. Taste.

8
THE BEAST: TIME MANAGEMENT

In a perfect world, the first 4 to 5 hours will be the busiest part of your shift. Why? You have 1 to 6 initial shift assessments to complete, the most medications to pass, and you are not familiar with your patients. Let's also pretend you have received a less than stellar report. Now you need to also figure out the plan of care for your patients.

All this action requires the dreaded words: Time. Management.

For the purposes of this chapter, let's refer to time management as *the beast*. This does not happen overnight, and from my experience, it is the most frustrating part of your new gig.

I get it. You've been a rock star high performer your whole life (me too). You told your manager in your interview that you are a fast learner, which is no doubt the truth (me too). You've never failed at anything (wellllll, kinda). The list goes on.

You are entering a new world, and all of this is about to change. And speaking from experience, this is the largest pill to swallow (like K-Dur big). We will get you through it.

I'll let you digest that for a second. Would you like that crushed and mixed with pudding?

TAME THE BEAST

Learn a Suggested Nursing Routine
Each floor will be different, but this is imperative for your success. Remember when I told you to figure out the nursing "flow" of your unit? If I am mentioning it again, it is that important.

Learn the routine/pace on the unit by observing the 7 Ws:
1. **When** most transfers happen
2. **When** most discharges happen
3. **When** nurses take breaks
4. **When** most physicians do rounds
5. **When** most medications are due
6. **Which** part of charting takes the most time
7. **What** the charting requirements for the floor are

Now take what you have observed and make a "perfect world" timeline for your day.

Example Timeline

0630–0645: Get assignment. Look up patient labs/read 1 physician note

0645–0655: Shift update/huddle (whatever you call it)

0655–0730: Hand-off

0730–0745: Fill in gaps needed to complete patient picture

0745–1130: 5 patient assessments & notes charted & all AM meds passed

1030–1200: Patient rounding (check-ins), discharge surge

1200–1300: Miscellaneous tasks & afternoon med pass

1300–1330: Lunch

1330–1400: Charting

1400–1600: Patient rounding, more discharges, miscellaneous tasks, charting

1600–1800: Expected transfers, evening meds, charting

1800: Final patient rounds before shift change

1850: Hand-off

Now, a couple of things to note. This is a timeline for the *perfect* nursing shift. Do perfect nursing shifts exist? I have yet to see one in my day, and I have learned to expect the worse.

So why do I bother mentioning this? As a new nurse, you need a plan. You need to set planned expectations and *assume the worst is going to happen to you.* Develop the habit of ensuring your assessments are charted and meds are passed by 1130 each day. Why? Because even if you miss the 1130 target by 1 hour because of unforeseen emergencies, you are still caught up on your charting. By doing this, you will *never* get in the habit of charting at the end of your shift, which always results in your staying after shift change to catch up.

What Can You Cluster?

Clustering is a survivalist strategy. If you can learn to cluster your care, you will master taming *the beast.* What does this mean?

Here is a scenario: You are looking up labs on your patient early in the shift. Suddenly, you get a call from the nursing assistant telling you there is tube feed all over your patient and that he needs a linen and gown change. This patient also has pain medication due, and you noticed that his IV fluids were running low during report. You *finish* writing down the patient's labs and then look at his medical record to determine if anything besides the pain medication is due. You see that the patient has 4 daily medications due in 30 minutes.

Think critically about this. It is going to take you around 20 minutes to change the patient. By the time you finish the gown change, the medications will be due. If you do not bring the pain medicine into the room, you will be late on the patient's pain medication. You learned in report that he is very particular about the time he receives his pain medication.

Here's What You Do
- Run and get an extra set of sheets and an extra pad for the bed just in case you are walking into a tube feed massacre.
- Pick up IV fluids on your way to the Pyxis.
- Pull the 4 medications due in 20 minutes.
- While at the Pyxis, also pull the patient's pain medication. (Remember: typically, you have 30 minutes to administer a narcotic once you pull it.)
- Enter the patient's room and explain you are going to give him his pain medication before you clean him up (wink: he will appreciate this).
- While you are changing the patient, you can do a thorough skin assessment.
- Change his sheets. During the linen change or once finished, do your efficient patient assessment.
- Now change the IV fluid bag out and pass his daily medications.
- While he is taking his meds, chart his assessment in the room.

Look at what you just did, you savvy nurse, you. You just passed pain medications, cleaned up a giant mess, gave your AM medications, and completed your assessment in 30 minutes.

Badda-bing. Badda-boom.

Don't Drop What You're Doing Unless It's an Emergency
Notice how I told you to first *finish* writing down your patient's labs when you got that phone call? Most new nurses immediately drop what they are doing every single time they receive a phone call. Don't do that. Not everything is an emergency. In your new profession, seconds and minutes count. *Finish what you are doing; otherwise, you will have to come back and complete the task you left.* Stopping what you are doing each time the phone rings opens you up to making mistakes or forgetting the task at hand.

Patients can wait 2 minutes to use the restroom while you finish a note. They can wait 4 minutes for pain medication while you finish looking up their labs. They can wait 10 minutes for their discharge paperwork while you empty a Foley catheter. If you drop everything you are doing anytime someone needs something, I promise you will spend your day bouncing back and forth, forgetting what you started, and making more people upset in the long run.

Unless it is an emergency, it can wait! If a patient can't breathe, stop what you are doing and get the heck in the room. If a patient's blood pressure is tanking, stop what you are doing and get the heck in the room. If a patient is unresponsive, stop what you are doing and get the heck in the room. Get the drift?

Hone Your Assessment Skills
Take that beautiful 30-minute head-to-toe assessment and cut the time in half at first. Yikes! I know! Give yourself 15 minutes to complete the assessment and set a timer. At first, you will be taking only a few patients, so 15 minutes per patient will be possible. This gives you an opportunity to get great at your assessment skills.

As you move through orientation and begin to increase your patient load, aim to safely shave off patient assessment time. This is a marathon, not a sprint. What happens when you spend too much time in one room? You will be behind for the rest of the day. The beginning of your shift is the sole predictor of the type of day you will have, and you better start the day with goals in mind.

Table 1 depicts target assessment times to improve time management as you increase your patient case load.

TABLE 1. Target Assessment Times			
Patient Load	Assessment Time	Med Pass Time	Total Time Spent
1 patient	20 minutes	20 minutes	40 minutes
2 patients	15 minutes	20 minutes	70 minutes
3 patients	10 minutes	15 minutes	75 minutes
4 patients	10 minutes	15 minutes	100 minutes
5 patients	8 minutes	12 minutes	100 minutes

Let me mention that this is not a one-size-fits-all. You may have an emergency or a very unhappy patient that requires more attention and time.

You might look at Table 1 and think that this is not possible. At first, it will not be. Do not set unrealistic expectations for yourself. However, it does give you a target to strive for and will prevent you from spending too much time in one patient's room, which is a very common problem for new nurses.

Learn the Art of Delegation

Remember when I said to respect the nursing assistants? Learning to delegate does not mean that you do not respect them. It means that you understand how to professionally and practically tame *the beast.* If a patient asks for a cup of ice when you are already headed toward the nutrition room to grab some pain medication, cluster your care and grab both. Do not send the nurse's aid to do this task. You will make enemies quickly, new nurse friend.

Now, if you're tied up in a patient room giving medications and another patient needs to be toileted, it is appropriate to delegate this task to the aid if he has the time. Remember, you have 1 to 6 patients, but he could have 8 to 20.

> A quick note to the new nurse who worked as an aid during school:
> Your role has changed, and you worked very hard to get where you are. You cannot handle it all. You are not superhuman. If you could, nursing assistants would not be employed.
> Ya'll hear me?

If you spend too much time completing tasks that could be delegated to an aid, you will get behind and you will not be capable of taming *the beast.* Take some advice from someone who learned this the hard way.

Prioritize. Prioritize. Prioritize.

It's very easy to decide to check on a patient who is short of breath first before you bring another patient pain medication. Prioritizing isn't always as straightforward as the bathroom versus chest compressions. That's what makes it so difficult during your first couple of months on the job.

One question I am asked frequently is how to prioritize who to assess first. I wish there was an easy answer, but there is not. Every day, every patient, every unit is consistently inconsistent. Buttttt, ask yourself the list of questions following, and it should help you tame *the beast*.

Priority Questions

Q: Is everyone stable? If the answer is *no,* get the heck in that patient's room!

Q: Who seems to be the "busiest" patient? Busy means various things. Lots of meds. Might be going downhill soon. Just likes attention. If everyone is stable and happy, I start my day in the easiest patient's room (independent, least amount of meds) and finish with the busiest (most medications, total care).

Q: Are there any medications due *right now* for anyone? What is the med? Is it time sensitive? If you have a time-sensitive med that can be given quickly with other medications, try clustering care for that patient first.

Q: Is anyone going to procedure? When are they going to procedure? What is left to be completed before they go (consents, antibiotics, CHG bath)?

Q: Does anyone have discharge or transfer orders? Does the house need beds? Your charge nurse or preceptor will know the answer to this. It will guide you on how quickly you need to get the patient out.

Q: Do you have any open beds? Is someone being admitted to that room soon? Is a patient already there waiting to be admitted?

All prioritization requires you to ask yourself a million questions to get to the correct order of priority. It is yet another skill that comes with time. I hope this helps you begin to understand the basics.

At first, you will find it impossible to tame *the beast*. I am not going to lie. But each day you will work a little harder and a little faster, and one day you will get there. I promise. It may take 4 to 6 months, but *the beast* can and will be tamed. Even on the craziest of shifts, you will leave on time and have eaten lunch to boot if you take this chapter seriously enough.

9
GIVING REPORT

Organizations around the country have shifted toward bedside shift report. If your organization does not do bedside shift report, I think you will see that this change is coming sooner rather than later.

Regardless of whether you do report inside or outside the room, you can quickly become a *boss* at your hand-off.

Basic Report Etiquette

- Be prepared.
- Know pertinent labs and patient history. *Pertinent* is the key word here. It is 2018, new nurse friend, and no longer relevant that your patient had an appendectomy in 1946.
- Don't bounce around, lose your train of thought, or frequently interrupt the other person.
- Paint a concise clinical picture.
- Give your report from head to toe in order of what you see.
- Report is not designed so that you can check all the boxes and fill in all the blanks on your report sheet. Every patient is different, and you could waste major time trying to search for information that is not relevant to that patient's care.
- Your patient rooms are a reflection of your nursing care. As the off-going RN, always round on each of your patients an hour before shift change. Use the last patient

round to tidy up rooms, administer pain medication, toilet patients, and complete any pending tasks. It is disrespectful to the next shift to make them walk into multiple patients with uncontrolled pain, needing to pee, soiled linen, and meds that were due 4 hours ago. There is no excuse for this. *You can and will do better than this.*

Shift happens! Because nursing is a 24/7 continuum of care, there will be times you will be late on action items and you must pass on tasks to the next shift. This is OK, but should not become a regular pattern. For orders that are received during shift change, it is typically the oncoming nurse's responsibility to handle. If there is a scheduled medication that was due 4 hours prior, kindly ask the off-going nurse to handle that before she leaves. Be kind. We're all in this together.

If you blank during report, start at the patient's head and work your way down the body in order.

Report Flow Using Anatomical Basics
Admitting Diagnosis⇨
Code Status⇨
Relevant History & Labs⇨
Head⇨
Chest⇨
Stomach⇨
Bladder⇨
Bowel⇨
Legs⇨
Skin⇨
IV⇨

Pain ⇨
Important Shift Events

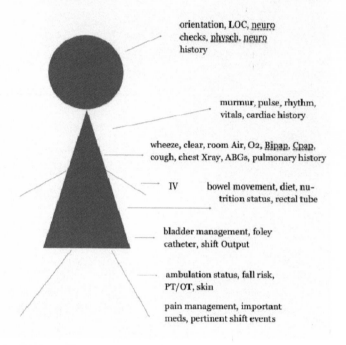

Figure 1. Report Flow

10
PAGING AN MD

When I was on orientation, I *hated* calling doctors. I felt stupid and wanted to crawl into a corner after each call. The reality is this:

It. Stinks. At. First.

You will be asked questions you inevitably don't know the answers to. Someone will yell at you. You will fumble your words. And all of these things you will get over. Quickly.

So here's the deal. Follow these dos and don'ts. It's not fail proof, but will at least help you reach boss status quicker.

Do
- Give the physician the patient's name and *concise* reason the patient was admitted. Fifty percent of the time they are taking the call for another provider and will need a small background on the patient.
- Get to the point quickly—*Quickly*, I said.
- Know your darn vital signs. There is no excuse not to have a current set of vitals when paging a physician. This includes the patient's blood glucose if it could be relevant in the least bit. Why not have it just in case?
- Ask yourself what you want to get out of the phone call. Are you calling to notify the doc of a patient change? It is OK to give him a heads-up about his patient. C.Y.A. Nine times out of 10, the doctors will appreciate it. Other times, they yell at you.

- Do you need orders? Think Ryan Gosling screaming at Rachel McAdams in *The Notebook*. What do you want? What do you want? You're welcome.
- If it helps, seclude yourself (if you can) in front of your patient chart. If you can have the information available, you will be ready for anything the doctor asks you. If that is not an option, write down everything you think the doctor could ask you when she returns your call.

Don't
- Be afraid to voice that you are concerned. Remember that nursing "gut" we talked about earlier? It's real. Telling doctors you think something is wrong even though you cannot pinpoint it is OK.

> **A little note here:**
> If you are going to tell the doctors that you think something is wrong, you must state *why* you think something is wrong. Is the patient more lethargic than before? Is her blood pressure significantly different than earlier? It doesn't matter what you want to communicate (to a degree), but you need to paint a picture for the docs over the phone.

- Wait for the physician to ask. That is frustrating for them. If you know you are going to need a K+ replacement, you best know the patient's potassium. If you know you are going to need blood pressure medication, you best know the patient's trending pressures. Ya'll hear me?
- Don't jeopardize patient safety because you are afraid to call or you are afraid of being yelled at. You didn't think that one was coming, did you? WWFD? We have

the most important job in the world—to protect our patients. The end. If you make that the reason behind everything you do, things become a lot easier.

11
YOUR FIRST CODE

On my second day off orientation, I heard the patient's monitor alarming while I was charting in his room. I was on a telemetry floor at the time. I turned to find my patient slumped over in bed and unresponsive. I calmly walked to the side of his bed. When I did not feel a pulse, I casually hit the code button above the bed.

Then I froze.

I did not start chest compressions. I did not do anything, in fact, but stand there in what I felt was the closest thing I have ever experienced to paralysis. It felt like my heart was literally pounding outside of my chest. My vision was blurry. My hands began to cramp up. I couldn't speak.

I vaguely remember someone pushing me out of the way because I was essentially useless. There was a doctor screaming at me to tell him about the patient.

A big-girl nurse walked over to me and instructed me to clench my fists and push them away from my body. Then repeat. Imagine me decerebrate posturing if you will. I know you know what that NCLEX word means.

So, there I was looking as if I were decerebrate posturing in the middle of a code. Ridiculous. But, you know what, new nurse friend? It worked. It released the adrenaline that was paralyzing me. My heart began to climb back inside its cavity, my vision straightened out, and I could move again.

I owe that big-girl nurse my patient's life. She taught me how to tame my adrenaline, which is no easy feat.

Role Play

There are two different roles you will play as a nurse during a code. If you are a bystander, your activities are going to differ than if you are the primary nurse.

TABLE 2. The 2 Roles During a Code	
Primary RN	**Just Wanna Help or Found Patient Down**
Start compressions if you find your patient down pulseless unless he is a DNR, which you better know, new nurse friend!	Start compressions if you find a patient down pulseless unless you know for certain the patient is a DNR.
Push the code button.	Push the code button.
Verify the patient's code status.	Verify the patient's code status.
Once the team arrives, stop compressions and let someone else take over.	Take over chest compressions for someone.
Learn to unfreeze yourself.	Grab the crash cart if someone hasn't already.
Do not run away. Only you know details about the patient that could save his life.	Be a bouncer; regulate entry into the room.
Be ready to spout off labs, pertinent patient history, procedures, trends, changes.	You can never have enough flushes. Go get 15 and hand them to someone in the room.
You can assist with meds if you are ACLS certified. Just be available for questions.	Go round on the primary nurse's other patients.

During orientation, your preceptor will be there to assist you. Remember that you are not alone! Insert yourself wherever you can in a code blue to gain more experience. The first time you do chest compressions might be traumatic, but the next time you will know what to expect.

12
OWN. LEARN. REPEAT.

So, here's the deal. You have just joined the best tribe in the world. Nurses are the most solid and trustworthy people in the world. We have each other's backs. Always. No matter what.

Yes, here comes the *but.*

We are human.
  We are busy.
    We are *really* busy.
      We have more to do than the time to do it.

Because of all this, we make mistakes. We forget to document an assessment. We have a patient fall. We lose patient belongings. We feed an NPO patient. We administer the wrong dose. ... The list goes on. We do all these things despite our best attempts to protect our patients.

> **WWFD?**
> When you make a mistake, recognize that you are only human. Assume responsibility like the boss you are and own it. Flo attributes her own nursing success to making no excuses! After you own it, learn from it. Promise me that you will learn from it. Mistakes have the magical power of turning you into a better nurse if you learn and embrace them.

13
C.Y.A.

I just got finished telling you we are human, and that we all make mistakes.

Always.
Always.
Always.

Verify the Information You Receive

If you have a heparin drip going at 1300 units/hr, verify the last PTT with your own eyes and review the protocol. It does not matter if the nurse before you told you what it was.

If you have just received a patient from the ER, and she told you that the patient has no wounds, do a skin assessment anyway.

If you are coming on shift and you hear that your patient was more altered during the night, go look at the patient *together*.

If you are coming on shift and you are told that a patient has NS running at 125 ml/hr, you better verify that NS is truly hanging and review the order with the nurse going off shift.

I just listed four instances that happened to me during my first month on the job. Were they intentional? Heck no! But they happened, and I learned to verify information I was told the hard way.

Each patient, each unit, each nurse, and each specialty is unique. Always verify.

14
ASK FOR FEEDBACK

This one is simple.

At the end of *every* shift, ask your preceptor to tell you what you did well and what you could improve on. This opens the door for constructive criticism and gives you real-time feedback on your progress.

I carried this into my nursing practice once I was off orientation. To this day, I ask myself what I did well and what I could have done better. It keeps me honest with myself and makes me a better nurse.

This reflection practice also gives you a chance to reflect on the amazing things you have done for your patients or fellow nurses. So often we downplay the crazy-stupid-awesome things we are doing for people. Pat yourself on the back every once in a while, nurse friend! You deserve it.

15
FEEL THE FEELS

Orientation is a weird rite of passage. No, this does not involve older nurses eating you alive. It is where you are humbled each and every day. You are scared. You learn and forget and are told again. Nursing orientation is the steepest learning curve out there, as far as I am concerned. Soooo ... Just feel the feels, ya'll! Okay?

Cry it out. Laugh it out. Scream it out. You do you.

How to Feel the Feels
- Acknowledge the emotion you are feeling in that particular moment.
- Name it. Is it joy, love, anxiety, terror, humor, sadness, compassion?
- Embrace it; don't fight it.
- Take a moment.
- Move forward.
- On your way home, repeat this sequence.

16
BE FLEXIBLE

I saved this token of virtue for last because it might be the most important.

Be. Flexible.

You've just entered the hardest and most demanding profession on the planet. The hours are grueling. The pay is typically peanuts for the magnitude of responsibility we carry with us every day. Patients can be downright disrespectful. Some are dangerous; others are kind. You can get hugged, kicked, punched, slapped, and loved all in the span of 2 hours.

Manage your expectations and be flexible. Your assignment may change midshift. You may be called in unexpectedly. You may have an entire patient assignment on droplet precautions. You may get floated to another unit. You may have a patient death and have an admit waiting for you in your next room.

Maybe ...
- Your assignment changed because your coworker got punched by a patient.
- You got called in unexpectedly because the unit is short staffed.
- All of your patients are on precautions because there is a community outbreak.

- You get floated to another unit because they don't have any nurses with the skill set to take a particular patient.
- You may have an admit waiting for you because the safest place for that patient to be is in your care.

Flexibility is required for you to succeed. Try to understand the bigger picture. If you can't, I promise someone making those decisions does.

17
STILL WITH ME, SUNSHINE?

So here we are. At the end of my laundry list.

We have all been standing right where you are and remember the feelings all too well. It is my hope that this book has given you ideas to help you navigate your new adventure, and brought you one step closer to Bey' status.

Becoming a nurse is not for the faint of heart. You will experience miracles and beauty. Pain and joy. Faith. Fear. Sadness. Love. Your journey will be one of a kind, yours to hold close to your heart or share with the world.

You are being initiated into one of the most sacred and magnificent tribes on the planet. This tribe is comprised of superheroes in scrubs who often endure the wildest of circumstances to protect the healing of mankind. As your fellow nursing soldiers, we believe in your success and will be here with you every step of the way.

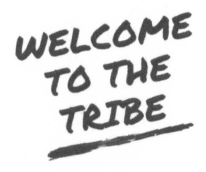